Glute P7-EOS-213

You have just been told that you have celiac disease or dermatitis herpetiformis (DH). With this new found knowledge, you can take the first steps in changing your lifestyle for a better and healthier you. You will finally be able to leave your symptoms and suffering behind you by adhering to a treatment that involves no medications, no side effects and no surgical procedures. Even if you have "asymptomatic" celiac disease, the long term health benefits of a gluten-free diet are great. All you have to do is cut wheat, rye and barley out of your diet. The word "diet" usually invokes thoughts of self-denial, but we are here to tell you that a gluten-free diet does not mean the end of beloved treats, monotonous and boring meals or the sacrifice of nutritional value.

People who do not currently suffer from symptoms may develop serious complications down the road if they do not adhere to a gluten-free diet. The good news is that a gluten-free diet is not as daunting as it sounds and with proper instruction you will be able to make a smooth transition into your new lifestyle.

So how do you completely banish unsafe foods without becoming overwhelmed? We wrote this guide to help you navigate the gluten-free life with ease, confidence, and lots of enjoyment. After using this guide for a while, you will find that selecting gluten-free foods and recognizing potential problem foods can be easy. You'll also see that a gluten-free diet can be rich and varied, offering plenty of delicious choices.

Cutting out wheat, rye, and barley does not mean the end of satisfying, healthy, and exciting meals!

The fact is, most foods are perfectly safe for you. A luscious bit of steak, a juicy pear, crunchy sugar-snap peas, or a baked sweet potato topped with a dollop of butter will never trigger celiac disease complications. You should be wary of processed foods made with wheat, rye or barley. Coatings, sauces, breaded items, and gravies are often made with flour – although they don't have to be. A good rule of thumb is the plainer the food the better.

Gluten-Free Basics

The gluten-free diet includes a plethora of options. You may be surprised at the number of naturally gluten-free foods you already eat on a regular basis. Meats, poultry, fish, fruits, vegetables, legumes, and dairy products that are in their natural or unprocessed state are all safe. In terms of starch: rice, corn, potato, oats, yucca, buckwheat, quinoa, millet, and teff are all safe. They do not contain the same protein sequence that wheat, rye, and barley have. Oats may be contaminated by gluten. There are more details on this later in the guide.

Here is a basic list of safe and toxic starches. Refer to the Grocery Shopping section for a complete guide.

Gluten-Free Replacement Choices
Available as flours, grains as well as in pastas,
baked goods, crackers and snack choices.

The items in **bold** are healthier choices (they
contain more fiber and nutrients). All flours and
grains **must** be labeled gluten-free (except rice).

Amaranth

Arrowroot

**Buckwheat (purchase only buckwheat
labeled gluten-free)**

Cassava

Coconut

Corn

Corn grits

**Cornmeal (preferably whole grain,
enriched cornmeal)**

Cornstarch

Flax

Legumes

Mesquite

Millet

Montina (Indian rice grass)

Nuts

**Oats (purchase only oats labeled gluten-
free; see section on oats)**

Popcorn

Potato (preferably sweet potato)

Quinoa

Rice (preferably enriched white rice, whole grain brown rice or wild rice)

Sorghum

Soy

Tapioca

Teff

Yam

Yucca

Toxic

Wheat (all forms including kamut, semolina, spelt, triticale)

Oats (unless labeled gluten-free)

Rye

Barley (including malt)

Brewer's Yeast

Reading Labels

In The United States

According to the Food Allergen Labeling and Consumer Protection Act (FALCPA), food manufacturers must disclose if a product contains protein from one or more of the top eight allergens (peanuts, tree nuts, soy, fish, shellfish, milk, eggs, and wheat). This must be listed on all product labels including foods, dietary supplements, and vitamins.

Gluten-Free Living

Each allergen must be listed by its "common name"—for example, "durum" would be listed as "wheat." Allergens in flavorings, colors, or incidental additives must be listed in accordance with these requirements as well. Therefore, if a food or ingredient contains wheat, in any form, it must be noted on the label. It could be listed in parentheses after the food, i.e. "soy sauce (soybeans, wheat, salt)" or on the bottom of the label as "this product contains wheat." Incidental additives, which include the flour used to dust the pan, conveyor belt, etc. must also be listed.

Currently, foods regulated by the United States Department of Agriculture (USDA) are not required to list the common allergens in the foods they regulate, although most do. The USDA regulates protein based food products including meats, poultry and egg products (this also includes processed meats such as sausage, pepperoni, beef jerky, lunch meats, bacon, etc). All meat, poultry and eggs in their natural, unprocessed state are gluten-free. Many of the companies that produce processed meats label their products gluten-free (refer to grocery shopping section). If a company does make a gluten-free claim, check for an allergen claim (ex. Contains milk/egg/soy). If a company makes an allergen claim and wheat is not identified, then the product should be safe to eat. If a processed meat is not labeled gluten-free and does not have any allergen information on the food label, check the ingredients. If it contains starch, modified food starch or dextrin, contact the company to make sure it is gluten-free.

In the future, the FDA plans to enact even more stringent food labeling laws in the United States. The FDA intends to set the standard of 20ppm as the upper limit for a food to be considered gluten-free. It will also require periodic testing of the product by state of the art techniques. However, wheat starch hydrolysates, which can be used in glucose syrups, caramel color, dextrin and maltodextrin have been given permanent exemption status stating that they already contain under 20ppm gluten and therefore do not have to disclose the ingredients. They are considered safe.

Outside the United States

Different standards exist in different countries. Codex Alimentarius is a commission set up by the World Health Organization (WHO) and the Food and Agricultural Organization (FAO) to develop international food standards and guidelines. The Codex standard for foods for special dietary use for persons intolerant to gluten was updated in 2008. This standard applies to foods for special dietary uses that have been formulated, processed or prepared to meet the special dietary needs of people intolerant to gluten. Gluten-free foods must not exceed 20 mg/kg of gluten. Low gluten or limited gluten (20-100 mg/kg) are not gluten-free and are not acceptable.

Additives:

These additives are generally safe.

Artificial color and flavor
Baking powder
Baking soda
Caramel color
Citric acid
Dextrin
Hydrolysed soy protein
Maltodextrin
Modified food starch
Mono and diglycerides
Monosodium glutamate (MSG)*
Natural color and flavor
Soy, soy protein (tofu)
Soy lecithin
Vanilla, vanillin, artificial vanilla, vanilla
   extract
Vinegar (**NOT** malt vinegar)
Whey

Products

Trade names are used selectively. The lists are not exhaustive. Some products are used as examples.

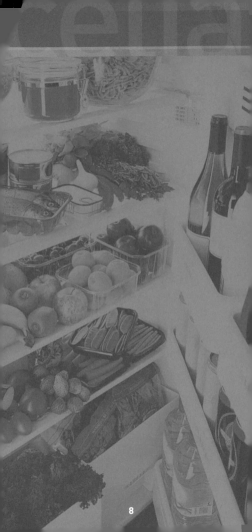

Getting Started

Many questions and fears exist. Remember that many of the foods you have in your kitchen cupboard and fridge are already gluten-free. This guide will help you sort it all out.

Naturally Gluten-Free Foods

Dairy

Cheese (except beer cheese and ale cheese)
Ice Cream (most are safe–read label. No cookie dough, cookies & cream, or brownie flavors)
Milk
Plain Yogurt (most fruit yogurts are safe, but read label)

Fruits, Vegetables

Canned Fruits and Vegetables (not all are safe–read label)
Fresh Fruits and Vegetables
Frozen Fruits and Vegetables (without sauce)

Meats & Alternatives

Beans, Legumes, Nuts, Seeds
Deli Meat (most are safe–read label and/or speak to manufacturer)
Eggs
Hummus
Meats, Poultry, Fish (unprocessed)
Nut Butters (most are safe)

Getting Started

Fats and Oils

Butter/Margarine
Salad Dressings (most are safe—read label)
Vegetable Oils
Vegetable Spray (not baking spray)

Sauces, Seasonings
Condiments that may contain gluten and **must** be checked include BBQ sauce, soy sauce, marinades, and sauces

Mayonnaise
Mustard (most are safe—read label)
Ketchup
Pickles, Olives, Relish
Spices

Things to Replace

Breads
Cereals
Cookies
Crackers
Pastas

Make sure to always read labels carefully. You will soon realize that there are a lot of things you can eat!

Remember wheat-free is **NOT** gluten-free

Cohabitation Survival/Cross Contamination

Here are some tips to help you avoid cross-contamination:

- Cutting board (designate as gluten-free or well cleaned between uses.)
- Colander (designate as gluten-free to keep your gluten-free pasta gluten-free.)
- Toaster (pop up toaster must be dedicated gluten-free.)
- Toaster oven (can be shared but foil must be used to prevent cross-contamination.)
- Separate containers or squeezable bottles for butter, mayonnaise, peanut butter, and anything you dip into.

Remember to color code them so they are easy to identify–have fun. Think of this as a way to restock your kitchen basics.

- Clean all counters and cutting boards carefully before preparing gluten-free meals or snacks.
- Clean all utensils, grills, dishes, pots and pans carefully before using them.
- Store all gluten-containing products in separate labeled containers. It may help to put bright stickers on foods that are to remain gluten-free (e.g. margarine, peanut butter, butter, cream cheese, etc.)

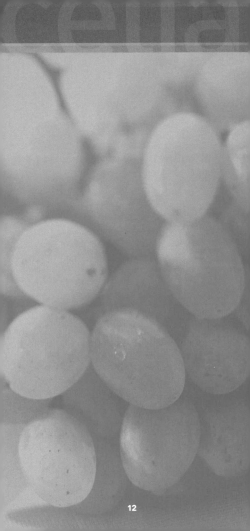

Gluten-free foods may be found in a variety of places:

- Go through your cupboards at home... you will find many staples that are safe on the gluten-free diet (e.g. ketchup, mayonnaise, peanut butter, etc.)
- Basic foods such as meats and alternatives, fruits and vegetables, dairy products and condiments can be found in any grocery store
- Local health food stores, gourmet type grocery stores and even many grocery store chains often contain a variety of gluten-free foods
- Look for organic or natural food sections
- Gluten-free foods can be ordered online directly from the company

Grocery Shopping Points to Remember:

- Always read food labels
- Wheat-free does not mean gluten-free
- When in doubt do without
- Remember that food items in bulk bins cannot be guaranteed gluten-free due to possible contamination issues

We have created a list of gluten-free foods. Please be advised that ingredients can change and that you MUST read food labels. This list does not include all gluten-free foods. If you find foods in the grocery store that do not contain gluten in the ingredients or that say gluten-free...go ahead and try them!!!!

Grocery Shopping

Items marked with an * denote that the item is either Kosher gluten-free or the company produces some, if not all, Kosher gluten-free products. Please refer to manufacturer's website to verify which items are Kosher.

Baby Foods

> Beech Nut (not all are safe–read label)
> Bella Baby*
> Happy Bellies (gluten-free ONLY)
> Heinz (gluten-free ONLY, see website for list)
> Petite Select
>> Arroz Con Pollo*
>> Mango Jamba*
>> Organic Baby Cuisine*
>> Shepherd's Pie*
> Tasty Brand (gluten-free ONLY)
> Toddler Health

Bagels

> Ener-G Foods*
> Enjoy Life*
> Food For Life Baking Co.*
> Gluten-Free Bagel Company
> Glutino
> Joan's GF Great Bakes, Inc.
> Kinnikinnick Foods, Inc.
> Udi's

Bakeries (dedicated gluten-free)

> Cause You're Special
> Celiac Specialties LLC
> Chébé Bread
> Ener-G Foods
> Enjoy Life

Grocery Shopping

Everybody Eats
Foods By George
Gillian's Foods
Gluten-Free and Fabulous
Gluten-Free Bagel Company
Gluten-Free Creations Bakery
Glutino*
Joan's Gluten-Free Great Bakes, Inc.
Josef's Gluten-Free*
Katz Gluten Free*
Kinnikinnick Foods, Inc.
Mariposa Baking Company
Miller's Gluten-Free Bread Co.
Mr. Ritt's Bakery
Patsy Pie
Schär
Shabtai Gourmet*
Silly Yak
Sunstart Bakery
The Grainless Baker
Three Dogs Gluten-Free Bakery
Udi's
Whole Foods

Baking Chips

Enjoy Life
Hershey's
Nestle
   Chocolate Chips
   Peanut Butter
Tropical Source
   Semi Sweet Chips

Baking Mixes (gluten-free ONLY)

1-2-3 Gluten Free
   Biscuits*

Brownie Mix*
Cake Mixes*
Muffins & Quickbreads*
Rolls*
Scrumdelicious Cookies*
Sugar & Spice Pan Bar Mix*
Sugar Cookies*
Allergy Free Foods
Amazing Grains
Andrea's Fine Foods
Arico Foods*
Arrowhead Mills*
Authentic Foods*
Barkat
Muffin Mix*
Betty Crocker (gluten-free ONLY)*
BiAglut
Bisquick (gluten-free ONLY)
Bob's Red Mill*
Breads From Anna*
Cause You're Special
Celiac Specialties
Celimix
Celinal Foods
Chébé Bread
Cherrybrook Kitchen*
Choices Best Rice Bakery
Dowd & Rogers
El Peto
Ener-G Foods*
Farmpure Foods
Food-Tek
Gifts of Nature
Gillian's Foods
Gluten-Free Bagel Company

Gluten-Free Creations Bakery
Gluten-Free Essentials
Gluten-Free Naturals*
Gluten-Free Pantry*
Glutino*
Heavenly Mills*
King Arthur (gluten-free ONLY)
Kinnikinnick Foods Inc.
Kokimo Kitchen
Miss Roben's
   Gluten-Free Soft Pretzel Mix*
   Gluten-Free Frosting Mix*
   Mock Gluten-Free Graham Cracker Mix*
Namaste Foods*
Nature's Own Bakery
Orgran*
Pamela's Products
Paneriso/Kingsmill
Really Great Foods
Ruby Range
Schär
Shiloh Farms
Sylvan Border Farm
The Really Great Food Company
Tom Sawyer

Baking Powder – All Safe

Baking Soda – All Safe

Barbeque Sauces

   Bone Suckin' Sauce*
   Buffalo Wild Wings Sauces
     Blazin
     Caribbean Jerk

Honey BBQ
Hot
Mango Habanero
Medium
Mild
Parmesan Garlic
Spicy Garlic
Sweet BBQ
Wild (not Asian Zing or Teriyaki)

Cattlemen's

Dinosaur BarBQ
Habanero
Regular

Kraft
Bull's-Eye
Chick'n Rib
Garlic
Hickory
Original
Sweet & Sour
Thick'n Spicy

Lea & Perrins
Marinade for Chicken
Traditional Steak Sauce
Worcestershire Sauce

Mr. Spice (several types & flavors)

Bars

Alpsnacks
Andi Bars
Bakery on Main
Gluten-Free Granola Bars*
Balance Pure
Bliss Bars
Bumble Bars

Almond
Awesome Apricot
Cashew
Chai
Cherry Chocolate
Chocolate Chip
Chunky Cherry
Hazelnut
Lushus Lemon
Mixed Nuts
Original
Tasty Tropical
CoFresh Snack Foods Ltd. (not all are safe—read label)
Comfort Bars*
Ener-g
Enjoy Life Bars*
EnviroKidz Snack Bars
Extend Bar*
    Delight Snack Bars
General Mills
    Nut Crunch
Genisoy Bars (not all are safe—read label)
Glenny's
    Brown Rice Marshmallow Treat*
Gluten Free Café
    Chocolate Sesame Bar
    Cinnamon Sesame Bar
    Lemon Sesame Bar
Glutino*
Good 'n Natural
Go Raw
Gorge Delights
    Blueberry Pear*
    Cranberry Pear*
    Pear*

Strawberry Pear*
Gourmet Guru Sesame Serenity Bars
Ian's
Apple Pie Go Bars*
Kind Fruit & Nut Bars
Kookie Karma
Lara Bars*
Leda Nutrition
Logia Bible Bars
Elijah's Fire Chocolate Treat*
Jacob's Ladder*
King David's Cranberry Nut*
Noah's Nuggets*
Seeds of Samson*
Luna Protein Bar
Mrs. May's Trio Bar*
Met-Rx High Protein Bars (not all are safe–read label)
Nogii Bar
NuGo Free
Carrot Cake*
Dark Chocolate Crunch*
Dark Chocolate Trail Mix*
Nugo Nutrition
Omega Smart Bars
Organic Fiber Bar
Orgran (fruit-filled bars)
Oskri Bars
Perfect 10 Bars
Potent Foods Organic Maca Bar
Prana Bars
Apricot Goji*
Apricot Pumpkin*
Coconut Acai*
Purefit Gluten-Free Protein Bars*
Quest Protein

Raw Revolution Bars*
Soy Joy
The Simply Bar
Think Thin (not all are safe—read label)
Trio Bars
Whole Foods Market Organic Honey
Roasted Snack Bars
Wings of Nature*

Beans

Beverages

Alcohol
Champagne
Cordials
Distilled Alcohol (gin, rye, rum, vodka, whiskey)
Sherry
Wine
Beer (gluten-free ONLY)
Bard's Tale Beer Company
Golden Sorghum Lager
Budweiser
Redbridge
Dogfish Head Tweason'ale
Green's Gluten Free Beers
Lakefront Brewery
New Grist
New Plant St. Peter's Sorghum
Ramapo Valley Brewery
Honey Beer*
Toleration
Coffee
Regular & decaffeinated (check label on flavored coffee or coffee drinks; may be flavored with malt)

Gatorade
Juice (most are safe—read label)
Soda
Tea (check label on flavored, herbal or tea drinks; may be flavored with malt)

Biscotti (gluten-free ONLY)

Pamela's

Breads & Bread Products (gluten-free ONLY)

Breads
Canyon Bakehouse
Ener-G*
Everybody Eats
Food For Life Baking Co.
Bread*
Brown Rice Tortilla*
Garbo Gluten-Free
Sport Bread*
Sun Bread*
Toast Bread*
GlutenOut
Heaven Mills
Joan's GF Great Bakes, Inc.
Josef's Breads*
Katz Gluten-Free
Kinnikinnick Foods, Inc.
Miller's Gluten-Free Bread Co.
Rudi's Gluten-Free Bakery
Schar
Whole Foods
Breadsticks
Glutino Food Group
Challah
Heaven Mills*

Katz Gluten-Free*
Kosher Naturals Gluten-Free Bakery*
English Muffins
Foods By George
Joan's GF Great Bakes, Inc.
Kinnikinnick Foods Inc.
Frozen Bread (gluten-free ONLY)
Against the Grain
Ener-G
Enjoy Life Food
Everybody Eats
Foods By George
Glutino
Joan's GF Great Bakes, Inc.
Kinnikinnick Foods, Inc.
Nu-World Foods Flatbread
Sherri's Cheese Rolls
Frozen Breadsticks (gluten-free ONLY)
Chébé Bread
Pita Bread
Heaven Mills*
Gluten-Free Pita

Bread Crumbs

Amaranth Bread Crumbs
Gillian's
Holgrain*
Ian's
Kinnikinnick Foods, Inc.
Nu-World Foods
Orgran
Shabtai Gourmet*
Shavit's Nutri Source*
Soynutbutter
Cornflake Crumbs*
Tortilla Crumbs*

Bread Mixes

Bread Mixes
Breads From Anna*
Cause Your Special
Celinal Foods
Chebe
Really Great Foods
Kinnikinnick Foods, Inc.
Tastes Like Real Food

Breakfast Meats

Al Fresco
Armour Brown 'N Serve
Jimmy Dean
Jones Links & Patties (not all are safe–read label)

Broth & Bouillon

Campbell's
Herb-Ox
Imagine
Organic Beef Flavored Broth
Organic Beef Flavored Stock
Organic Chicken Stock
Organic Free Range Chicken Broth
Organic Low Sodium Beef Flavored Broth
Organic Low Sodium Beef Flavored Stock
Organic Low Sodium Chicken Stock
Organic Low Sodium Free Range
Chicken Broth
Organic Low Sodium Vegetable Broth
Organic No Chicken Broth
Organic Vegetable Broth
Organic Vegetable Stock
Kitchen Basics

Maggi
Osum*
Pacific
Redi-Base*
Shelton's
Streits*
Swanson

Brownies

Eragrain*
Foods By George

Cake

Frank's Gourmet Mouse Cakes*
GlutenOut
Heaven Mills Cakes
  Brownie Cake*
  Chocolate Kokosh*
  Cinnamon Kokosh*
  Cupcakes*
Lean On Me Gluten-Free*
New Harvest Naturals Gluten-Free Bakery
  Pound Cake*
Shabtai Gourmet
The Lite-ful Cheesecake

Cake & Dessert Toppings

Betty Crocker Chocolate Sprinkles
Betty Crocker Sweet Toppings Carousel
Mix Sprinkles
Hanan's Products*
Hershey's Hot Fudge & Caramel Sauce
InstantWhip Topping*
Rich's Non-Dairy Whip Topping*
Tofutti*

Grocery Shopping

Canned Chicken
Swanson
Valley Fresh

Canned Fish
Clams, Mackerel & Oysters
Ace of Diamonds
Beach Cliff
King of Oscar
Roland
Rubenstein's
Snow's
Underwood
Great King
Salmon*
Sardines*
Tuna*
Tuna – All Safe

Canned Fruit – All Safe

Canned Olives – All Safe

Canned Vegetables
Plain Canned Vegetables
(check if in sauce)

Cereals (hot & cold) (cereals must be labeled gluten-free)

Cold Cereal
Ancient Harvest
Quinoa Flakes*
Arrowhead Mills
Corn Flakes
Maple Buckwheat Flakes
Maple Corns

Bakery on Main
  Granola
Barbara's Bakery
  Brown Rice Crisps*
  Corn Flakes*
  Honey Rice Puffins*
Celiac Specialties
  Granola
Cereal Vit Gluten-Free Cereals
Enjoy Life Foods
  Cinnamon Crunch
  Granola
  Very Berry Crunch
EnviroKidz
  Amazon Frosted Flakes
  Gorilla Munch
  Koala Crisp
  Orangutan-O's
  Panda Puffs
Erewhon
  Aztec Crunch Corn & Amaranth
  Brown Rice Cream*
  Cornflakes*
  Crispy Brown Rice*
  Rice Twice*
General Mills
  Chocolate Chex
  Cinnamon Chex
  Corn Chex*
  Honey Nut Chex
  Rice Chex*
  Strawberry Chex
Health Valley
  Blue Corn Flakes
  Corn Crunchums
  Rice Crunchums

Heartland's Finest
  CerO's
Kay's Naturals
  Apple Cinnamon*
  French Vanilla*
  Honey Almond*
Kellogg's Rice Krispies (gluten-free ONLY)
Nature's Path
  Corn Flakes
  Corn Puffs
  Honey'd Corn Flakes*
  Mesa Sunrise
  Rice Puffs
  Whole O's
Nu-World Foods
  Amaranth O's*
  Original & Peach
  Amaranth Cereal Snaps
  Cinnamon, Cocoa, & Original
  Puffed Amaranth Cereal*
Perky's Natural Foods
  Perky O's*
  Nully Flax
  Nutty Rice*
Post
  Coco Pebbles
  Fruity Pebbles
Seitenbacher
  Muesli
  Cornflakes
Trader Joe's
  Granola
Udi's Gluten-Free Granola

Hot Cereal (must be labeled gluten-free)
Arrowhead Mills

Gluten-Free Rise and Shine
Gluten-Free Yellow Corn Grits
Bob's Red Mill
Gluten-Free Buckwheat Groats
Gluten-Free Corn Grits
Gluten-Free Creamy Brown Rice Cereal
Pocono Cream of Buckwheat
Wolff's Kasha

For complete information on Gluten-Free Oats, see alphabetical Oat listing in Grocery Shopping section.

Cheese (read ingredients, no beer cheese or ale cheese)

Cheese Sauce

Kraft
Macaroni & Cheese Sauce Packet
(do not use the macaroni)
Prego Low Carb Cheese Sauce
Trader Joe's
Alfredo Sauce
Velveeta

Chicken Nuggets (not all are safe—read label)

Applegate Farms
Bell & Evans Gluten-Free
Ian's

Chips (no composite chips like Pringles)
Plain chips are safe, read label for flavored varieties.

Bloom's*
Danielle Foods Gluten-Free Chips
Doritos (not all are safe—read label)

Flamous Brands Falafel Chips*
Foods Should Taste Good
Frito-Lay
Glenny's Popcorn Chips*
Guiltless Gourmet*
Kay's Naturals
    Better Balance Protein Gluten-Free Chips*
    Chili Nacho
    Crispy Parmesan
    Lemon Herb
Kettle
Krispy Crunch Puffs*
Lay's* (see website for gluten-free list)
Lunberg Rice Chips*
Mediterranean Snack Food Company
Mr. Krispers*
Myrnas Skinny Chips
Perach Rice Cakes*
Pinnacle Gold
    Baked Potato Chips*
    Veggie Chips*
Plocky's Gluten-Free Hummus Chips*
Riceworks*
Snyder's of Hanover (gluten-free ONLY)
UTZ (not all are safe–read label)*
Wise (not all are safe–read label)*

Cookies (gluten-free ONLY)

Aleias
Andean Dream
Arico*
Aunt Gussie's*
Barkat
    Chocolate Cream Filled Gluten-Free
    Wafers*

Lemon Cream Filled Gluten-Free
  Wafers*
Cherrybrook Kitchen
Dr. Lucy's
Enjoy Life Food*
Eragrain
  Chocolate Chunk*
  Oatmeal Raisin*
E-Z Gourmet
Glenny's*
Glow Gluten-Free
Glutano*
Glutino
Golden Taste*
Good Eatz
Health Valley
Heaven Mills*
Hoffner Gluten-Free Cookies*
Ian's
Joan's GF Great Bakes, Inc.
Josef's Gluten Free*
Kinnikinnick Foods, Inc.
Leda Nutrition
Lieber Passover Cookies
Lilly's Gluten-Free Cookies*
Maggie's Gluten-Free Goodies*
Mariposa
Midel
  Arrowroot Cookies*
  Chocolate Chip
  Ginger Snaps*
  Mini Chocolate Chip
  Pecan
  Pecan Shortbread
Nana's (gluten-free ONLY)*

Natural Nectar (gluten-free ONLY)
Nutritious Creations (gluten-free ONLY)*
Orgran*
Pamela's
Pandaroos Delights
Patsy Pie
Schar
Shabtai Gourmet*
Shibolim*
Streits*
Sunstart Bakery
Sweet Christine's
Sweet Deliverance
Whole Bakers
Whole Foods

Frozen Cookie Dough (gluten-free ONLY)
Gluten-Free Pantry Ready Bake
    Buckwheat Raisin
    Chocolate Chip

Crackers (gluten-free ONLY)

Amy Lyn's Original Flax Thins
Bi-Aglut
Bloom's Corn Cake Thins & Rice Cake Thins*
Blue Diamond
Carole's Soycrunch
Crunchmaster•
Eden Foods
Edward & Son Rice Crackers
Feng Shui Rice Crackers*
Foods Alive*
Glutano*
Glutino Crisp Bread Crackers
Goldbaum's Natural Food Co.
Holgrain*
KaMe

Kay's Naturals
Mary's Gone Crackers*
Mediterranean Snack Food Company
Mr. Krispers*
Mrs. Crimbles Gluten-Free
Nut Thins by Blue Diamond
Orgran*
Real Foods Corn Thins
Schar
Snack Pac Oriental Rice Crackers*
Wellaby's

Deli – Sliced Meats

Applegate Farms
Boar's Head
Black Bear (not all are safe–read label)
Carl Buddig
Dietz & Watson
Di Lusso
Honeysuckle White
Hormel 100% Natural
Hormel Natural Choice
Jenni-O Turkey Store
John Morrell
Kroger's Store Brand
Kunzler (not all are safe–read label)
Oscar Mayer (not all are safe–read label)
Sugardale (not all are safe–read label)
Thumann's

Eggs

Egg Beaters (not all are safe–read label)
Fresh Eggs
Just Whites

Extracts – All Safe

Flours (flours **MUST** be labeled gluten-free)

Amaranth
Arrowhead Mills
    Blue Corn Meal
    Brown Rice Flour
    Buckwheat Flour
    Millet Flour
    Organic Flax Seed Meal
    Soy Flour
    White Rice Flour
    Yellow Corn Meal
Arrowroot
Bean
Buckwheat
Chickpea
Coconut
Corn (not corn bread mix unless specified as gluten-free)
Manischewitz*
Mesquite
Millet
Montina
Nut
Oat
Potato
Quinoa
Rice (white, brown, wild)
Sorghum
Soy
Tapioca
Teff

Frozen Donuts/Cinnamon Rolls (gluten-free ONLY)

Celiac Specialties

Conte's
Everybody Eats
Kinnikinnick Foods, Inc.
Nutralicious Natural Bakery, Inc.
 Wheat-Free with Soy Yogurt Glaze
 Wheat-Free Cinnamon with Soy
 Yogurt Glaze

Frozen Entrees & Dinners

Amy's (gluten-free ONLY)*
Angel's Touch*
Ayoob Storable Foods*
China Mehadrin*
Conte's
 Ravioli
DePumas Pasta
Delimex
 Chicken Taquitos
Dr. Praeger's
 California Veggie Burgers*
 Gluten-Free Broccoli Littles*
 Potato Littles*
 Spinach Littles*
 Sweet Potato Littles*
El Burrito Food Products
 Soy Taco*
 Soyrizo*
Everybody Eats
Feel Good Foods Dumplings
Garden Lites*
Get Healthy America*
GlutenFreeda
Gluten Free Café
 Asian Noodles
 Fettucini Alfredo

Homestyle Chicken & Vegetables
Lemon Basil Chicken
Pasta Primavera
Savory Chicken Pilaf
Glutino*
Nutritious Creations Beef Corn Dogs*
Olive Valley Gluten-Free Falafel Sticks*
Organic Bistro
S'Better Farms*
Beef Gluten-Free Corn Dogs*
Chicken Ballontine*
Chicken Fingers*
Chicken Sicilano*
Chicken Szechwan*
Chicken Wings*
Schwan's
Beef Tamales
Star Lite Cuisine
Starfish Gluten-Free Battered Seafood
Sunshine Burgers
Veggie Burgers

Frozen Fries

Ian's
Ore-Ida (not all are safe—read label)*

Frozen Macaroni & Cheese

Amy's (rice pasta ONLY)
Glutino

Frozen Pizza (gluten-free ONLY)

Amy's (made with rice crust ONLY)
Foods By George
Glutino
Kinnikinnick Foods, Inc.

Nature's Highlights
Sherrie's

Frozen Pizza Crust (gluten-free ONLY)

Barkat
Foods By George
Glutino
Kinnikinnick Foods, Inc.*
Nature's Highlights
Schar
Sherrie's
Whole Foods Market

Frozen Pizza Dough (gluten-free ONLY)

Gillian's Pizza Dough
Quejos

Frozen Waffles/Pancakes (gluten-free ONLY)

EnviroKidz Gluten-Free
Life Stream Gluten-Free
Van's Gluten-Free*

Grain Side Dishes (gluten-free ONLY)

Amaranth
Amazing Grains
  Montina
Ancient Harvest
  Quinoa
Arrowhead Mills
  Amaranth
  Buckwheat Groats
  Hulled Millet
  Quinoa
Bob's Red Mill
  Whole Grain Enriched Cornmeal
Buckwheat

Gogo Rice
  Quinoa Bowls
  Rice Bowls
Millet
Nu-World Foods
  Amaranth
Polenta
Potato
Quinoa
Rice (white, brown, wild)
  Lundberg Family Farms Rice &
  Rice Blends
  Only Oats Oat & Rice Mixes
  Tambo Bamba Rice Mixes
  Trader Joe's Rice Trilogy
Risotto
Sorghum

Gravy Mix

Glutino
Gravy Master
Imagine
  Organic Beef Flavored Gravy Heat & Serve
  Organic Turkey Gravy Heat & Serve
Kitchen Bouquet
Orgran

Hoisin Sauce

Premier Japan

Honey – All Safe

Ice Cream (not all are safe–read labels)
(not cookie dough, cookies and cream, or
brownie flavors)

Baskin-Robbins

Ben & Jerry's*
Breyer's*
Carvel*
Coconut Bliss
Country Fresh*
Dairy Queen
Edy's
Goldstone (not all flavors)
Good Humor*
Haagen-Dazs
Klein's Real Kosher*
Machmirim*
Nestle
  Dibs*
Nogürt*
Red Mango
Rice Dream Non-Dairy
  Carob Almond
  Cocoa Marble Fudge
  Neopolitan
  Orange Vanilla
  Strawberry
  Vanilla
  Vanilla Bites
So Delicious
  Creamy Fudge Bar*
Soy Dream Non-Dairy
  French Vanilla
  Green Tea
  Mint Chocolate Chip
  Mocha Fudge Swirl
  Vanilla Fudge Swirl
Tasti D-Lite (not all flavors)
Tempt*
Turkey Hill
Turtle Mountain*

Grocery Shopping

Ice Cream Cones

Barkat*
Cerrone
Gedilla*
Tovli

Ice Tea Mixes

Crystal Light
Lipton
Nestea

Icing (not all are safe—read label)

Betty Crocker
Cherrybrook Kitchen
Duncan Hines
Pillsbury

Indian Sauces

Geeta's (not all are safe—read label)
Taj Ethnic Gourmet
Calcutta Masala
Punjab Saaq Spinach Sauce
Wild Thymes*

Jams, Jellies, Marmalades – All Safe

Ketchup – All Safe

Marinades & Sauces

Al Arz Tahini
Bone Suckin'
Chunky Salsa*
Hiccupin Hot*
Hot Mustard*
Hot Sauce
Original Flavor*

   Seasoning & Rub*
   Thick Sauce*
   Yaki
  Emeril (not all are safe—read label)*
  Haddar
   Barbecue Sauces*
   Duck Sauces*
  IMO Foods Thai Curry Paste*
  Jack Daniel's EZ Marinader
   Garlic & Herb Variety
  Mikee
   All Purpose Chinese Marinade with Garlic*
   Apricot & Peach Duck Sauce*
   Buffalo Style Wing Sauce*
   Cajun Style Sauce*
   Fra Diavlo Sauce*
   Garlic Stir Fry & Spare Rib Sauce*
   Lemon Butter Dill Sauce*
   Lemon Butter Herb Sauce*
   Sweet & Sour Duck Sauce*
   Sweet Chili Sauce*
  Osem*
  Terra Sol
   Citrus & Spice Steak Sauce
   Habanero Honey Mustard
   Peru de Chile Chipotle
  Wild Thymes*

Marinara Sauce (most are safe–read label)

Marinated Vegetables

Matzo

  Barkat Gluten-Free Matzo Crackers*
  Doctor Katz's Oat Gluten-Free Matzos

Lakewood Bakery Gluten-Free Matzo*
Yehuda Matzos (gluten-free ONLY)

Mayonnaise – All Safe

Meat (all unprocessed meat, fish and chicken is safe)

Milk – All Safe

Milk Substitutes

Almond Dream
  Original Enriched
  Original Enriched Unsweetened
Haddar
  Coffee Whitener
MimicCreme*
Pacific Almond Milk*
Rice Dream*
  Classic Carob
  Classic Original
  Classic Vanilla
  Enriched Chocolate
  Enriched Original
  Enriched Vanilla
  Heartwise Original
  Heartwise Vanilla
  Horchata
  Supreme Chocolate Chai
  Supreme Vanilla Hazelnut
Soy Delicious*
Soy Dream
  Classic Original
  Classic Vanilla
  Enriched Chocolate

Enriched Original
Enriched Vanilla
Enriched Refrigerated Original
Enriched Refrigerated Vanilla
Tempt Hempmilk*

Muffins

Eragrain*
Kosher Naturals*
Frozen Muffins (gluten-free ONLY)
Foods By George
Kinnikinnick Foods, Inc.
Whole Foods
Udi's

Mustard (most are safe—read label)

Nut Butters (most are safe—read label)

Nuts

Blue Diamond
Smokehouse Almonds
Bone Suckin'
Fire Dancer Jalapeno Nuts & Hot Nuts
Wine Nuts
Gefen Chestnuts*
Haddar Chestnuts*
Planters
Dry Roasted Peanuts
Trader Joe's
Chocolate Covered Almonds, Peanuts,
and Cashews
Whole Food Market (365 Brand)
Maple Pecans
Spicy Pecans
YumTee*

Oats

Studies have indicated that a moderate amount of gluten-free oats is safe for people with celiac disease. Before introducing gluten-free oats, there should be no gastrointestinal complaints and celiac disease should be well controlled on a gluten-free diet (as indicated by negative antibodies). Oats are high in fiber and may cause gas and a change in stool pattern. These symptoms should resolve in a few days. Adults with celiac disease should limit gluten-free oats to 1/2-3/4 cup dry rolled oats per day. Children should limit gluten-free oats to 1/4-1/2 cup dry oats per day. A small percentage of people with celiac disease do not tolerate oats. If symptoms of intolerance persist, contact your physician or nutritionist.

Oats

> Arrowhead Mills (gluten-free ONLY)
> Bob's Red Mill (gluten-free ONLY)
> Cream Hill Estates
> Farmpure Foods
> Gifts of Nature
> Gluten Free Oats
> Gluten Freeda
> Great Northern Growers
> Holly's Au Natural Oatmeal
> Legacy Valley
> Only Oats
> PrOatina

Oil Sprays (oil spray ONLY – not baking spray)

> PAM

Trader Joe's
Store brands are usually safe, read label

Oils – All Safe

Olives – All Safe

Pancake Mixes (gluten-free ONLY)

1-2-3 Gluten Free Buckwheat Pancake
Mix*
Arrowhead Mills
  GF P&W Mix
  Wild Rice P&W Mix
Authentic Foods*
Bob's Red Mill
Gluten-Free Pantry
Kokimo Kitchen
Namaste Foods
Only Oats
Pamela's
Sylvan Border Farms
Whole Foods Market (365 Brand)

Pasta (gluten-free ONLY)

Ancient Harvest (quinoa & corn bi-aglut)
Bi-Aglut
Bionature*
Conte
De Pumas
DeBoles
  Angel Hair Plus Golden Flax
  Gluten Free Rice Shells & Cheddar
  Rice Angel Hair Pasta
  Rice Fettucini
  Rice Lasagna
  Rice Pasta Plus Golden Flax

Rice Penne
Rice Spaghetti Style Pasta
Rice Spirals
Wheat Free Corn Elbow Style Pasta
Wheat Free Corn Spaghetti Style Pasta
Eden Foods
Everybody Eats
Gillian's Foods
Glutano
GlutenOut
Glutino
Goldbaum's*
King Soba Gluten-Free Ramen Noodles
Le Veneziane
Lundberg
Mrs. Leeper's
Nutrition Kitchen soy pasta*
Orgran*
Papadini Pasta*
Pastariso
Sam Mills Corn Pasta*
Schar
Seitenbacher
  Garden Ribbons
  Rigatoni
Solterra Foods
Streitz Passover Chow Mein Noodles*
Tinkyada (brown rice)*
Trader Joe's Brown Rice Pasta

Pasta Dishes (gluten-free ONLY)

Allergaroo
Orgran Gluten-Free Spaghetti with
Tomato Sauce

Pastry Mixes

> GlutenOut
> Orgran

Peanut Butter (most are safe—read label)

Pickles, Pickled Vegetables – All Safe

Pizza Crust Mix (gluten-free ONLY)

> Arrowhead Mills
>   GF Pizza Crust Mix
> Barkat*
> Chebe
> Domata Living Flour
> Garbo*
> Gluten-Free Pantry
> Rustic Crust

Popcorn (movie popcorn safe)

> Bachman's*
> Dale & Thomas*
> Golden Fluff*
> Ike & Sam's Kettle Corn*
> Indiana Kettle Corn*
> Jiffy Pop
> Jolly Time
> Kettle Corn NYC
> Newman's
> Orville Redenbacher
> Pop Secret

Prepared Meals

> A Taste of Thai
> Go Picnic
> My Own Meal

      Beef Stew*
      Chicken & Black Beans*
      Chicken Mediterranean*
      My Kind of Chicken*
      Old World Stew*
    Perdue Short Cuts

Pretzels (gluten-free ONLY)

    Barkat*
    Ener-G*
    Glutino*
    Kay's Naturals*
    Nu-World Foods Amaranth Snackers
    Osem
    Snyder's of Hanover (gluten-free ONLY)

Puddings (most are safe–read label)

Relish – All Safe

Rice Cakes

    Hain
    Health Valley
    Lundberg Family Farms
    Organic Brown Rice Cakes
    Quaker (most are safe–read label)

Salad Dressings (most are safe–read label)

Salsas – All Safe

Salty Snacks

    Mini Pops Inc. Popped Sorghum Grain
    Ricepod Gluten-Free Snack Mix
    The Good Bean Roasted Chickpea Snacks

Sausages/Hot Dogs (smoked sausage & fat-free hot dogs may not be safe—read label)

> Agri Star*
> Applegate Farms
> Boar's Head
> Coleman's
> Hebrew National (not all are safe—read label)
> Hillshire Farms
> Kahn's Beef Franks
> Nathan's (not all are safe—read label)
> Oscar Mayer (not all are safe—read label)
> Sabrett
> Thumann's

Seafood (all unprocessed seafood is safe)

> Frozen
> > Fjord King*
> > Seagate*
> > Shinder's*
> > Starfish Gluten-Free Battered Seafood
> > Stoller Fisheries*
> Gefilte Fish
> > A&B*
> > Freund's*
> > Oneg*
> > Pike and White*
> > Shinder's*
> > Stoller Fisheries*

Soups

> Amy's*
> > Kitchen Organic Cream of Tomato (regular or light sodium)
> Baxters Food Group (not all are safe—read label)

Campbell's
  Chunky Chicken with White & Wild Rice
  Select Harvest (not all are safe–
  read label)
  Split Pea & Ham
Gluten Free Café
  Black Bean
  Chicken Noodle
  Cream of Mushroom
  Veggie Noodle
Health Valley Organic (not all are safe–
read label)
Imagine (most are safe–read label)
Kettle Cuisine
King Soba Miso
Manischewitz*
Pacific (not all are safe–read label)
Progresso
  Black Bean
  Chicken & Rice
  Chicken & Wild Rice
  Cream of Mushroom
  Lentil
  New England Clam Chowder
  Potato Broccoli & Cheese
Tabatchnick Soups (not all are safe–
read label)
Wild Veggie Gluten-Free Soup

Soups (Instant/Meal in a Bowl)

Fantastic Whole Foods
(not all are safe–read label)
  Goodman's
  Onion Soup Mix*
Haddar Passover Soups

Beef Soup Mix*
Chicken Soup Mix*
Mushroom Soup Mix*
Onion Soup Mix*
Potato Soup Mix*
Lipton Onion Soup Mix*
Nile Spice Soups (not all are safe–read label)
Simply Asia
Thai Kitchen Rice Noodle Bowls
(not all are safe–read label)

Sour Cream – All Safe

Soy Sauce (not all are safe–read label)

Haddar*
Kikkoman (gluten-free ONLY)
LaChoy
Osem Chinese Style Soy Sauce*
Super 8
W.Y. International Inc.

Spices (all pure spices are safe, for
"seasonings" or seasoning mixes–read label)

Spreads, Dips

Cream Cheese (most are safe–read label)
Hummus (not all are safe–read label)
Sabra*
Tribe*
Sour Cream Based Dips (not all are safe–
read label)
Tahini
Tofutti Spread
Yogurt Spread
Brummel and Brown

Sugar

All sugar & artificial sweeteners

Syrups – All Safe

Tamari Sauce

San J (wheat free)

Teriyaki Sauce

Haddar*
Premier Japan

Tofu

Mori-Nu*

Tortillas

La Tortilla Factory
Teff Wrap
Mission Corn Tortilla

Trail Mix

Carole Soy Crunch
Cinnamon Raisin*
Coconut*
Original*
Sesame*
Toffee*

Turkey (fresh, frozen, not self-basting)
(most are safe–read label)

Vanilla (most are safe–read label)

Vinegar – All Safe Except Malt Vinegar

Rice Vinegar (not all are safe–read label)

Vinegar – All Safe Except Malt Vinegar

> Rice Vinegar (not all are safe–read label)

Water

Yeast – All Safe Except Brewer's Yeast

Yogurt (not all are safe–read label)

> Brown Cow*
> Givat Goglite*
> Machmirim*
> Mahadrin Fit'n Free*

Nutritional Notes

Studies have shown that people on the gluten-free diet may not be consuming enough vitamins, minerals, and fiber. Gluten-free grains are not typically fortified with vitamins and minerals.

Iron

Iron is a mineral found in food. The body needs iron to make blood. Animal food sources of iron (e.g. red meat and poultry) are better absorbed than vegetable sources (e.g. spinach). To help improve iron absorption, consume iron containing foods along with foods rich in vitamin C (e.g. citrus fruits, red peppers, potato, turnip, brussel sprouts). The Dietary Reference Intake (DRI) for iron is 8 milligrams daily for men, approximately 15 milligrams daily for women, and between 7-10 milligrams daily for children. The DRI is increased to 27 milligrams daily for pregnant women and those who are lactating should have approximately 9-10 milligrams daily.

Grocery Shopping

Sources of iron include:

Amaranth Grain
Dried Fruits
Edamame
Enriched Gluten-Free Cereal
  (Rice Chex, Corn Chex, Kellogg's Gluten-Free
  Rice Krispies, Puffins Gluten-Free Multigrain,
  Post Fruity Pebbles, Post Cocoa Pebbles)
Enriched Long Grain White Rice
Fish
Green Leafy Vegetables
Legumes
Meat
Millet Grain
Montina Flour
Nuts & Seeds
Poultry
Quinoa
Quinoa Grain
Rice Bran
Sorghum Grain
Soy Flour (defatted)
Teff Grain & Flour

Folate

Folate is necessary for the production and maintenance of new cells. This is especially important during periods of rapid cell division and growth such as pregnancy. The Dietary Reference Intake (DRI) for folate is 400 micrograms. Adolescents and adults should consume 400 micrograms daily. The DRI is increased to 600 micrograms daily for pregnant women and those lactating should have 500 micrograms daily.

Sources of folate include:

- Banana
- Beef Liver
- Chestnut Flour
- Chicken Liver
- Chickpea Flour
- Enriched Corn Flour
- Enriched Long Grain White Rice
- Green Vegetables (peas, broccoli, brussel sprouts, collard greens, okra)
- Ground Flax
- Hazelnuts
- Legumes
- Millet
- Orange Juice
- Peanuts
- Sesame Seeds
- Soy Flour
- Sunflower Seeds
- Walnuts
- Wild Rice

Dietary Fiber

Dietary fiber is an important part of the diet. It helps to maintain normal bowel movements and has also shown to be beneficial in the prevention of chronic diseases such as certain types of cancer, diabetes, and heart disease. Most adults should consume approximately 30 grams of fiber daily. Children should consume approximately 20-25 grams of fiber daily.

Some tips to increase fiber:

Read food labels.
Almost all food labels display the amount of dietary fiber per serving. The package can claim "high in," "rich in" or "excellent source of" fiber if the product provides 5 grams of fiber per serving.

Start the day with a whole-grain gluten-free cereal.
Top with raisins, ground flax seed, bananas, or berries, all of which are good sources of fiber.

When appropriate, eat vegetables raw.
Cooking vegetables may reduce fiber content by breaking down some fiber into its carbohydrate components. When you do cook vegetables, microwave or steam only until they are al dente—tender, but still firm to the bite.

Avoid peeling fruits and vegetables.
Eating the skin and membranes ensures that you get every bit of fiber. Make sure to rinse all fruits and vegetables with

warm water before eating to ensure that surface dirt and bacteria have been removed. Also, keep in mind that whole fruits and vegetables contain more fiber than juice, which lacks the skin and membranes.

Eat liberal amounts of foods that contain unprocessed grains in your diet. Include products such as quinoa, millet, or buckwheat.

Add beans to soups, stews, and salads. Substitute legume-based dishes (such as gluten-free lentil soup, baked beans, or rice and beans) for those made with meat.

Keep fresh and dried fruit on hand for snacks.

Not all gluten-free grains and flours are good sources of fiber. Try to include high fiber whole grains in your diet.

Fiber Content of Gluten-Free Flours and Grains

0-5 grams fiber per 1 cup serving	5-10 grams fiber per 1 cup serving	10-20 grams fiber per 1 cup serving	20+ grams fiber per 1 cup serving
Arrowroot Starch	Potato Flour	Amaranth Grain and Flour	Buckwheat Bran
Corn Flour	Quinoa Flour	Bean Flours	Corn Bran
Cornstarch	Brown Rice Flour	Buckwheat Flour and Groats	Ground Flax and Flax Seed
Potato Starch	Soy Flour	Chickpea Flour	Mesquite Flour
Tapioca Flour Tapioca Starch	Teff Flour	Cornmeal	Montina Flour
White Rice Flour		Corn Flour (whole grain)	Rice Bran
		Legumes	
		Millet Flour	
		Nuts and Seeds	
		Quinoa	
		Sorghum	
		Soy Flour (defatted)	
		Teff	

Grocery Shopping

Personal Products

Any personal product that is used on the exterior of the body is safe because gluten is not absorbed through the skin. Shampoo, soap, make-up, lipstick, and cleaning products are all safe.

Bath Products

Laundry detergent, bath soaps, shampoos, conditioner, lotions and bubble bath are all safe because they are not ingested.

Medications and Supplements

All medications and supplements, both over-the-counter and prescription, need to be checked for gluten content. Although corn starch is most commonly used, wheat starch and other gluten based ingredients can be used as compounding agents.

Below are some common over-the-counter medications that we have identified as gluten-free. Check with the manufacturer or your pharmacist for your prescription medications. Also, refer to **www.glutenfreedrugs.com**.

Remember to always read labels!
Advil
Aleve
Allegra
Aspirin
Clarinex
Claritin
Ecotrin

Imodium
Lomotil
Motrin
Mylanta
Robitussin
St. Joseph Aspirin
Sudafed
TheraFlu
Tylenol

Vitamins

We suggest that you have your blood vitamin levels checked annually. To prevent vitamin and mineral deficiencies while on a gluten-free diet we recommend a gluten-free multivitamin. When choosing a vitamin it is very important that it is labeled **gluten-free.** It is equally important that the vitamin does not contain too much of certain vitamins/minerals. Do not take a B complex in addition to the multivitamin.

To prevent osteopenia and osteoporosis it is also important that your diet provides enough calcium and vitamin D. Most adults require 1000-1300 mg of calcium per day which can be achieved through diet alone or with supplements (or both). Dairy products provide calcium-speak to your dietitian about how to meet your calcium requirements. You will need at least 400 IU of Vitamin D a day to meet your requirement. We suggest having your vitamin D level checked annually.

Notes:

Grocery Shopping

Notes:

Notes:

There are Good Grains and Bad Grains

Safe Grains & Flours

- Amaranth
- Arrowroot
- Bean flours
- Buckwheat
- Cassava
- Chickpea flour
- Coconut flour
- Corn (popcorn, corn grits, cornmeal, corn flour, cornstarch, corn bran, corn niblets, corn on the cob)
- Flax seed
- Mesquite flour
- Millet
- Montina flour
- Nut flours
- Oats (gluten-free)
- Potato (flour, starch)
- Quinoa
- Rice (flour, brown rice, white rice, wild rice, rice bran)
- Sorghum
- Suy (flour, soybean)
- Tapioca (pearls, flour, starch)
- Teff
- Yams
- Yucca

Unsafe Grains

- Wheat in all its form, including kamut, semolina, spelt, and triticale
- Barley, including malt
- Rye

Glossary of Grains

Do not be intimidated by grains. They are easy to cook and just as delicious as our old standbys - be adventurous! Try one of the nutrient packed alternative grains and taste buds watch out! Grains can be used as hot or cold cereal, side dishes, in soups and stews, as flour for pancakes or in baked products.

Amaranth

Once a sacred food of the Aztecs, Amaranth has a corn-like aroma and woodsy flavor. It is best suited to porridge-type dishes and ground into flour for bread. High in protein, dietary fiber, iron, magnesium, zinc, calcium, and B vitamins.

Buckwheat

Also known as kasha if toasted, buckwheat is best recognized for its use in flour form for pancakes and soba noodles. This hearty grain can be used as a hot cereal, a side dish, in soups, stews and casseroles, or in salads and stuffings. It can also be used as a flour for baking, thickening, and in pancakes. Buckwheat is rich in high quality protein, magnesium, B6, dietary fiber, iron, niacin, thiamin, and zinc.

Millet

Millet is dry and airy when cooked with a little water and moist and dense when cooked with extra water. Bland in flavor, it readily takes on the flavor of foods it is cooked with. Millet can be served as a hot cereal or side dish and can also be used for baking instead of flour. High in protein and fiber.

Oats

Oats are highly nutritious and filled with cholesterol-fighting soluble fiber. They also have a pleasant, nutty flavor. Most of us are familiar with rolled oats, which are used as a hot breakfast cereal and cookie ingredient. Oatmeal is also commonly used in such foods as meatloaf (as an extender), breads, muffins, cookies, granola, muesli, stuffing, and pilaf. Oat flour may also be used as a thickener in soups and stews.

For contamination issues surrounding oats, please refer to the alphabetical oat listing in the Grocery Shopping section.

Quinoa

This is a native South American grain with a soft, crunchy texture. Quinoa boasts the highest nutritional profile of all grains – it's often called a "super grain." Quinoa contains higher quality protein than other grains and cereals. It is also high in iron, magnesium, B vitamins, calcium, and fiber.

Sorghum

Sorghum is somewhat neutral in flavor and easily absorbs other flavors so can be used in a variety of dishes. It is often eaten as a porridge, ground into flour, or even popped like popcorn. This grain is high in fiber and iron and has a relatively high protein content,

Glossary of Grains

Teff

Teff is a nutritious grain that can be used as a hot cereal, a side dish, in casseroles, or served cold as a salad. It can be used in place of flour to thicken sauces, and is also available as pasta. High in protein, calcium, iron, and B vitamins.

Wild Rice

Taste, aroma, size, and color depend on whether the rice is wild or cultivated, where it is harvested, and the processing method. Wild rice is high in dietary fiber, protein, potassium, and zinc. This grain may be used as a side dish.

Flour Substitutes and More

Flours from various beans are another great gluten-free baking ingredient. They add a variety of nutrients, give foods a fabulous texture and have a great nutty taste. Bean flours have higher protein content than standard rice flours and behave more like wheat flour in baking. The protein in bean flours allows baked products to develop proper structure and mouth feel.

Chickpea flour has a mild, sweet taste. It works really well in cookies, muffins, cakes, and quick bread recipes. It can also be substituted for regular flour in a one-to-one ratio without any further changes to the original recipe. There is no need for any other additives.

Lentil flour has a stronger flavor than chickpea flour. It is wonderful for making bread or pasta.

Glossary of Grains

Mesquite flour comes from the bean pods of the mesquite tree and can be dried and ground into flour to be used in a variety of baked goods. Mesquite features a sweet, nutty flavor and is rich in calcium, magnesium, iron, and zinc.

Montina flour has a rich wheat like taste and a hearty texture. This flour works best when used in darker baked goods. Montina is milled from Indian ricegrass and is high in both protein and fiber.

Sorghum flour is a wonderful high protein – high fiber flour. It works well in combination with chickpea flour in quick breads, cookies, and bars.

Gluten-Free Baking

When modifying a favorite family recipe, try the following tips:

Gluten-free flour mixes can be used on a one-to-one ratio with regular flour. Walk through the natural food section of your local grocery store to see if they carry any gluten-free flour mixes. Mixes can also be ordered online or found in health food stores.

To add moisture to the recipe, add extra fruits, or grated vegetables. Frozen blueberries, mashed bananas, applesauce, pureed pumpkin, grated carrots, dessicated coconut, yogurt, and sour cream all work very well.

To improve taste, add extra flavors such as cinnamon, vanilla, nutmeg, or your favorite spice.

Gluten-free flours must be stored in a tightly

sealed package and kept in the refrigerator or freezer.

Do not get discouraged! Be prepared to enjoy some of the recipes more than others. If a recipe does not turn out well, grind up the baked goods and use as crumbs for a pie crust for another recipe.

Xantham gum is a polysaccaride, a type of sugar or carbohydrate, that can be helpful with baking. It can be added to a recipe to prevent food from crumbling. Generally, you can use 1 teaspoon xantham gum per one cup of gluten-free flour. Flour mixes usually already have xantham gum and should not require additional amounts to be added.

Baked goods should be removed from the pan before they cool. Once out of the pan they can be eaten immediately or frozen to preserve them.

Most gluten-free baked goods (breads, muffins, bagels) taste better if they have been toasted or warmed before eating (cookies do not require additional heating).

Gluten-free cookbooks are helpful. Most provide information on the different types of flours used and the qualities in the various flours. There is no perfect replacement for wheat flour so most recipes combine different gluten-free flours.

Gluten-free oat flour is a nutritious flour that also works well in recipes as a substitution for wheat flour. If a recipe calls for 2 cups of wheat flour, use 1 cup gluten-free oat flour plus 1 cup gluten-free flour mix or 2 cups of gluten-free oat flour.

Grain Preparation Table

*Gluten-free broth or soup may be used as a substitution for the water to add flavor to the grain.

Grain	Amount of Liquid	Amount of Grain	Cooking Time	Uses
Amaranth	1 cup	1 cup	Simmer 7 minutes, let stand 5 - 10 minutes	Hot cereal
Buckwheat	2 cups	1 cup	Simmer 15 minutes	Hot cereal, side dish, casserole
Millet	1 1/2 cups	1 cup	Simmer 15 minutes, let stand covered 10 minutes	Hot cereal, side dish
Oats	1 cup	1/2 cup	Simmer 15 minutes	Hot cereal, binder for meatloaf
Quinoa	2 cups	1 cup	Simmer 10 - 15 minutes	Side dish, cold salad
Teff	2 cups	1/2 cup	Simmer 15 - 20 minutes	Hot cereal
Wild Rice	1 cup	1 cup	Simmer 30 minutes	Side dish, stuffing

Here are some great ways to introduce your new grains:

Citrus Buckwheat Pilaf

2 tbsp butter or oil
1/4 tsp oregano
1 cup whole buckwheat groats (hulled grain)
1/2 cup finely chopped pecans
2 cups stock; beef, chicken or vegetable
1/2 cup currants
2 tbsp chopped, fresh parsley
1 tbsp grated orange or lemon rind
Salt and pepper to taste

Preheat oven to 350°F (180°C).
Melt butter or oil in a large saucepan over medium heat.
Add buckwheat. Add stock, cover, and cook for 15-20 minutes or until most of the liquid is absorbed.
Add remaining ingredients except parsley.
Transfer to a greased 1-qt casserole dish, cover, and bake for 20 minutes.
Garnish with parsley.
Serves 6.

Millet & Teff With Squash & Onions

1 cup millet
1/2 cup teff grain
1 onion, diced
1 butternut squash (skin removed) cut into bite sized pieces
4 1/2 cups gluten-free chicken or vegetable broth
Salt & pepper to taste

Rinse millet and teff and add to a large pot
along with salt, onion, and squash.
Add 4 1/2 cups of broth to pot, mix ingredients.
Simmer, uncovered, for 20 minutes or until
all the water is absorbed.

Quinoa Black Bean Salad

1/3 cup quinoa
1 cup water
1 tsp olive oil
4 tsp fresh lime juice, or more to taste
1/4 tsp ground cumin
1/4 tsp ground coriander
1 tbsp finely chopped fresh cilantro
2 tbsp minced scallions
1-1/2 cups cooked black beans
(15 oz can, drained)
2 cups diced tomatoes
1 cup diced bell peppers
(red, green, yellow, or a mixture)
2 teaspoons minced fresh green chiles
Salt and pepper to taste
Garnish with lemon or lime wedges

Rinse the quinoa well in a sieve under cool
running water.
In a saucepan, bring the water to a boil.
Add the quinoa, cover, and simmer on low
heat until all of the water is absorbed and
the quinoa is tender, about 10 to 15 minutes.
Allow to cool for 15 minutes.
In a large bowl, combine the oil, lime juice,
cumin, coriander, cilantro, and scallions.
Stir in the beans, tomatoes, bell peppers,
and chiles.

Add the cooled quinoa, salt and pepper to
taste, and combine thoroughly.
Refrigerate until ready to serve.
Garnish with lemon or lime wedges.
Serves 4 as a side dish.

Tabouli

2 cups quinoa, cooked
1 cup chopped parsley
1/4 cup chopped scallions
2 tbsp fresh mint or 1 tbsp dried mint
1 garlic clove, pressed
1 tbsp basil
1/2 cup lemon juice
1/4 cup olive oil
Salt & pepper to taste
Mix quinoa, chopped vegetables, and spices
in a medium sized bowl
In separate bowl, whisk lemon juice, olive
oil, and salt and pepper.
Add oil mixture to quinoa mixture.
Refrigerate at least 24 hours and serve.
Serves 4 as a side dish.

Chicken Nuggets, Tenders, or Fish Sticks

1 lb Chicken breast (or flounder cut
into strips)
1 cup chickpea flour
1 cup crushed potato chips
1/2 tsp pepper (use white if color is
an issue)
1/2 tsp garlic salt
1/2 tsp oregano, crushed
1-2 eggs beaten

Heat oven to 400°F.
Lightly coat the bottom of a baking pan
    with oil.
Mix together the dry ingredients.
In separate bowl, beat the eggs.
Cut the chicken or fish into desired size
    and/or shapes.
Dip chicken or fish into the egg mixture and
    then into the dry mixture.
Place chicken or fish onto baking sheet and
    bake for 20 -30 minutes for chicken
    (depending on the size and thickness),
    and 8-10 minutes for fish.
Serves 4.

Socca (Chickpea Flatbread)

2 cups chickpea flour (about 8oz)
2 cups cold water
1/4 cup olive oil, plus extra for cooking
2 tsp chopped fresh rosemary
1/2 tsp kosher salt
1/2 tsp freshly ground black pepper

Combine all ingredients in mixing bowl &
    whisk until large clumps of flour are
    incorporated & mixture thickens slightly,
    about 5 minutes (do not overmix)
Cover and rest in the refrigerator at least
    1 hour.
Heat large nonstick pan over medium heat
    and add 1 tsp olive oil to coat pan.
Add 1/4 cup batter and quickly rotate the
    pan to spread evenly (so thin like a crepe).
Cook about 3 minutes or until slightly
    brown on edges.

Run spatula underneath to loosen socca
from pan and remove.
Repeat with remaining batter.
Season with freshly ground pepper and
serve.

Yellow Corn Arepas

2 lbs frozen corn kernels, thawed
1 1/2 cup whole grain enriched yellow cornmeal
9 oz mozzarella cheese, grated
2 tbsp milk
1 1/2 tbsp sugar
Pinch of salt

Coursely grind corn kernels using meat
grinder and place in mixing bowl.
Add cornmeal, cheese, milk, sugar, and salt.
Mix thoroughly with electric mixer.
Using a 1 1/2 or 3 inch mold, shape the
arepas.
Stack arepas on a lightly greased baking sheet
with parchment paper between layers.
Refrigerate for 30 minutes.
Cook arepas over low to medium heat until
golden brown, approximately 3 minutes.
Serves 4.

Meatballs
1 pound extra lean ground beef
1 egg
1 onion, diced
1 cup sherry
1 cup spicy ketchup

Preheat oven to 350°F.
Mix beef with egg and onion.
Place meatballs onto a baking sheet and
    cover with foil.
Bake in oven until brown, 20-30 minutes.
Remove meat from oven and remove excess
    fat by patting meatballs with a paper
    towel.
Mix sherry and ketchup in a small
    saucepan on the stove.
Bring mixture to a boil, stir, and reduce
    heat to a simmer.
Add meatballs to saucepan, cover, and
    simmer for 1-2 hours.
Serves 4.

A Note about Meatloaf and Meatballs:

Use oatmeal or buckwheat in place of the
    bread crumbs in your favorite recipe.
Add the egg, chopped vegetables, and
    spices as usual.

Hint If vegetables are not popular with your
family, try adding pureed carrots, green
beans, beets, and broccoli into the meatloaf.
The flavor of the meat masks the vegetables.

Glossary of Grains & Recipes

Cookies

Pick your favorite recipe and substitute chickpea flour for regular flour in a one-to-one ratio. For increased protein and fiber, use half chickpea and half sorghum flour.

Cookie Bars

Use regular recipe, but substitute flour.
Add oats, dried fruit, chocolate chips, nuts, or seeds to taste.
Bake in a 13 x 9 inch pan at 350°F for 20 to 25 minutes.
Cut into squares (freezes well).

Muffins and Quick Breads

Substitute the flour.
Again you can use just one or an easy combination of 1/2 chickpea and 1/2 sorghum flours or a gluten-free flour mix.
Add your favorite fruits, nuts, or other gluten-free add-ins.

Pie Crusts

Two options:
1) Ground nuts or nut meal
2) Gluten-free ginger snaps

Use either as it graham crackers.
Mix with shortening, brown sugar and a dash of gluten-free flour.
Press into pie pan.
Bake for 10 minutes at 350° F.
Fill with your favorite pie filling and enjoy!

Apple Crisp

4 cups peeled, diced apples
3/4 cup brown sugar
1/2 cup gluten-free oat flour
1/2 cup gluten-free oats
3/4 tsp cinnamon
1/3 cup margarine

Preheat oven to 375°F.
Spread apples onto bottom of ungreased
    baking pan.
Mix next five ingredients well.
Cover apples with mixture & bake until
    crispy (about 25 – 30 minutes).

Snickerdoodle Cereal Mix

1/4 cup sugar
1 tsp cinnamon
2 cups Cinnamon Chex cereal
2 cups Chocolate Chex cereal
4 cups air-popped popcorn
1/4 cup margarine

Combine cereals & popcorn in large
    microwave safe bowl.
Combine sugar and cinnamon in small bowl.
Melt margarine & pour over cereal mixture.
    Stir to coat.
Microwave mixture uncovered for 2 min-
    utes, stirring after 1 minute.
Sprinkle sugar mixture over cereal mixture
    and stir to combine.
Microwave 1 minute, then spread on large
    cookie sheet to cool.

Apple Bars

4 cups cinnamon Chex
2/3 cup chopped dried apples
1/2 cup sweetened dried cranberries
1 tbsp margarine
1/2 cup light corn syrup
1/4 cup packed brown sugar

Line bottom & sides of 8-inch square pan with foil. Spray with cooking spray.
Mix cereal, apples, and cranberries in large bowl.
Heat butter, corn syrup, and brown sugar in small saucepan, stirring constantly, until sugar dissolves and mixture comes to boil. Boil 2 minutes, stirring.
Pour sugar syrup over cereal mixture in bowl and stir to coat.
Press mixture firmly into pan & refrigerate 1 hour or until firm enough to cut.

Soft & Chewy Oatmeal Raisin Cookies

1/2 cup butter, softened
1/2 cup granulated sugar
1/2 cup firmly packed brown sugar
1 egg + 1 egg white
1/2 tsp vanilla
1 cup gluten-free flour mix
1/2 tsp baking soda
1 tsp baking powder
1/4 tsp salt
1 tsp cinnamon
1 1/2 cups gluten-free oats
1/2 cup raisins

Cream the sugars and butter until fluffy.

Add eggs one at a time and incorporate thoroughly.

Add vanilla and stir.

In separate bowl, combine dry ingredients (except oats).

Stir dry ingredients into creamed mixture.

Stir in oats and raisins, cover bowl and chill 2 hours.

Preheat oven to 350°F.

Roll dough into tablespoon sized balls and place at least 2 inches apart on parchment-lined cookie sheet.

Bake for 8 – 10 minutes, or until lightly brown.

Transfer to a cooling rack immediately.

Sorghum Cranberry Bread

1 1/2 cups grain sorghum flour
1 1/2 cups Montina Gluten-free flour mix
2 tsp xanthan gum (or gelatin)
2 cups granulated sugar
3 tsp cinnamon
1 tsp salt
1 1/4 tsp baking soda
4 eggs
2 cups applesauce
1/2 cup buttermilk
3 cups fresh cranberries
1 cup chopped walnuts
Course sugar

Preheat oven to 350°F. Lightly coat loaf pans with nonstick cooking spray.

Combine flours, sugar, cinnamon, salt & baking soda.

Separate eggs.

To egg yolks, add applesauce & buttermilk .
Beat well.

Gradually add dry ingredients to applesauce
mixture and beat just until combined.

Beat egg whites until stiff, but not dry, and
fold into batter.

Stir in cranberries & walnuts.

Transfer to prepared loaf pans, top with
course sugar.

Bake 45-55 minutes or until edges begin to
pull away from sides of pan
and toothpick inserted in the center
comes out clean.

Let stand 5 minutes and remove from pans
to cool on rack.

Tea Bread of Barmbrack

1 cup strong tea, hot
1/2 cup chopped mixed candied peel
1 cup raisins
1 cup brown sugar
1 cup gluten-free flour mix (eg. Montina)
1 tsp baking powder
1/4 tsp baking soda
1/4 tsp salt
1 egg, beaten

Pour hot tea over candied peel, raisins,
and sugar.

Let stand overnight.

Preheat oven to 300° F.

Beat eggs and add to fruit mixture.

Mix together dry ingredients and add to egg
and fruit mixture.

Pour into greased 9 x 5" loaf pan and bake
for 1-1/2 hours.
Remove from pan and cool.

Yummy Gluten-Free Chocolate Chip Cookies

2-1/4 to 2-1/2 cups chickpea flour
1 tsp baking soda
1 tsp salt
1 cup (2 sticks) margarine
3/4 cup granulated sugar
3/4 cup packed brown sugar
1 tsp vanilla
2 eggs
2 cups chocolate chips (or preferred mix-in)

Preheat oven to 375°F.
Combine dry ingredients.
Cream together margarine, sugars, and
vanilla.
Add eggs one at a time, beating after each
addition.
Gradually add flour mixture and stir in
chocolate chips or your favorite mix-ins
(raisins, dried cherries, dried cranberries,
etc).

Drop by spoonful onto ungreased cookie
sheet.
Bake for 9 to 11 minutes and transfer to
cooling rack immediately.

Alternatives

Cookie bars:
  Grease 13 x 9 inch pan
  Bake for 20 to 25 minutes

Create your own flavor or bar:
  Add dried cranberries, nuts, oats, seeds, or even substitute half of the butter with peanut butter. For a lower fat version, substitute 1/2 of the margarine with apple sauce.

Notes:

_____

_____

_____

_____

_____

_____

_____

_____

_____

_____

_____

_____

_____

_____

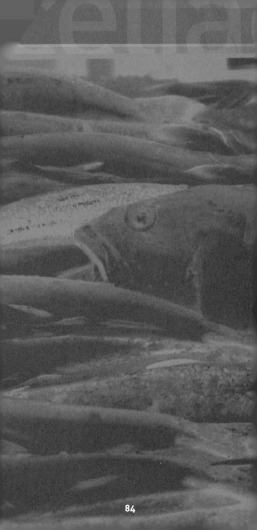

Restaurant Guidelines

Eating out can be a pleasurable experience, and following the gluten-free diet should not change that. While many places now have a gluten-free menu, you should not limit your options to those restaurants. It may take a little longer for you to decide what to order, but you can still eat a safe and delicious meal whether you're joining a last minute dinner date with friends, strolling through the streets in an unknown city, or going back to what was your favorite restaurant before your diagnosis of celiac disease. With the help of the tips below, we encourage you to make the most out of dining out anywhere!

Use the Internet. If you know your plans in advance, many restaurants now post their menu online allowing you to read through and choose items that may be safe for you.

Call ahead, especially if you are uncomfortable asking a lot of questions once you are at the restaurant. This alerts the chef that he/she will need to prepare a safe item. Remember to call at "off-hours", not during the middle of a lunch rush hour.

Always identity yourself as someone needing a special diet. Use a statement such as: "I have a food intolerance". Avoid the use of the terms "autoimmune disease" and "gluten" as these are terms not easily understood by the average restaurant server.

Restaurant Guidelines

Speak to manager, maître d' or chef. The key is to get your special needs conveyed to the chef or cook. If your waiter appears uninterested or unwilling to help, ask for the manager.

Ask specific questions (see list of questions below) about any menu items that could be deep fried or contain hidden gluten sources. Use a dining card to help the staff understand your special diet. If language is a barrier use language cards which can be found online.

Order simple dishes and ask for the sauce on the side or omitted altogether.

Ask about flour dusting. Even desserts that contain no gluten are often baked in a baking dish that has been dusted with flour.

Do not hesitate to send food back if not correct.

Be prepared to leave a restaurant if you feel your needs are not taken seriously.

Thank your server and leave a generous tip for good service.

Be a repeat customer to gluten friendly restaurants as they will try hard to please a regular guest.

Restaurant Guidelines

Questions to Ask the Server/Chef

Is there flour in this sauce?

Are there croutons on the salad?

What is in the BBQ sauce?

What is in the salad dressing?

Is the meat or chicken marinated? Check marinade.

Which foods are deep fried? Avoid foods cooked in shared oil.

Which of your dishes contain soy sauce?

Is there any flour, batter, or breading?

Are the noodles rice or wheat based?

Is the pan dusted with flour?

Is the tortilla 100% corn?

Are the corn chips deep fried?

Is this real or imitation seafood?

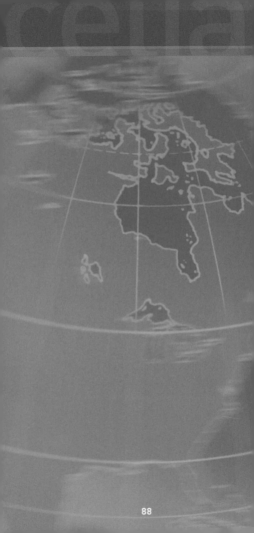

Plan Ahead

The most important thing is to plan ahead! Travel (international or domestic), dining out, or even a Sunday afternoon hike are all great opportunities to enjoy life – gluten-free. Celiac disease is very manageable. With some planning, you can eat safely when traveling by land, air or sea and maintain a nutritious, diverse, gluten-free diet once you reach your destination.

Traveling should not be a big deal. People may feel more comfortable about planning ahead. Especially if one is traveling by plane or train, you may be able to organize menus with different airlines or at least know in advance that none of the items offered are gluten-free. You can then bring your own food along. This may also apply to car travel in areas where gluten-free products are not available.

If possible, pack gluten-free food to bring with you when you travel. Good choices include peanut butter, tuna fish, crackers, cheese sticks, fruit, nuts, pretzels, bars, and trail mix. Even if you think you won't need it, delays or other unforeseen events could arise, leaving you hungry and without access to gluten-free food.

International Travel

Planning ahead with your physician is important and will help you reach your destination in a safe and enjoyable manner. You may need immunizations and medications depending on your destination, activities, length of stay, and health history. Most vaccines take time to become effective so consult with your physician several months prior to your trip. Try to do some reading on local food in the particular country or region you are traveling to. There may be some delicious gluten-free options available!

Domestic Travel

Consider shipping some food and snacks to the hotel ahead of time. Make sure that all packages are clearly marked and let the hotel manager know. Plan to have it couriered the day prior to your arrival. This will ensure that your favorite gluten-free foods will be ready and waiting when you arrive. If you will be changing hotels, have packages sent accordingly to each destination. This saves you from carrying a suitcase of gluten-free treats. However, if you decide to carry your food with you, as you nibble your way through your trip, you will give yourself more room for souvenirs.

Getting There

By Air (plane)

Although in-flight meal service is becoming less common, airlines that provide meals may offer a gluten-free option. All airlines require advanced notice so ask about the procedure when booking your flight and call to confirm a day or two before your trip. Always pack extra food that can be eaten if your gluten free meal is not provided or for your wait at the airport.

Peanut butter, gluten-free crackers or bars and dried fruit are easy to pack and should keep you full and satisfied for hours.

By Land (car, bus, train)

Traveling by car is easy. Pack a cooler or picnic basket and enjoy! Things that are easy to enjoy on long car rides include cheese, fruit, and packed sandwiches. Fast food chains often provide allergen information. If you do stop by a restaurant, ask questions or look for a brochure or listing with information.

Hiking & Athletic Activities

Hiking and backpacking are celiac heaven. There are many gluten-free meal replacement bars; trail mixes are a great high-protein gluten-free food and work well whether used as a mid-hike snack, post run nibble, or fueling up for a day on the slopes. Many rice bowls and vegetarian bowls/packets are gluten-free, lightweight, and just require boiling water for a delicious on the trail meal. Of course, don't forget the fresh fruit, plenty of water, and a good gluten-free chocolate bar for energy.

By Sea (cruise)

Several of the cruise lines now offer gluten-free meals. Some even bake their own gluten-free bread and rolls. Some cruises offer naturally gluten-free food as part of the buffet at every meal. As this varies from cruise to cruise, it's best to check ahead of time. Upon arrival, speak with the maître'd to let them know you'll need a gluten-free diet so they can offer advice and guidance throughout the trip.

For all travel, contact the hotel/resort/cruise ship where you will be staying to identify available resources. Find out what facilities the room has: is there a refrigerator, toaster, toaster oven, microwave, or coffee pot? If there isn't one in the room, would you have access to one? Once you know what is available, you know what types of goodies you can plan to bring, or have shipped to the site. Next, find out if there is a dining room in the hotel. Are meals included and can they provide for your diet? Calling ahead makes all the difference in the world. You will have peace of mind and the hotel/restaurant will be better prepared to serve you. It may be helpful for you to suggest gluten-free products with accompanying website information for easy ordering. With advance notice, hotel catering staff is generally receptive to providing gluten-free catering for special occasions, conferences, etc.

Dining

Eating out at restaurants should not be a big deal. You may feel more comfortable by planning ahead. This may involve calling ahead, looking at menus, or speaking with the maître'd. Some restaurants even have gluten-free menus online.

It may help to find gluten-free restaurants through the internet or local support groups. However, using gluten-free restaurants is not usually a necessity for the enjoyment of dining out. See Restaurant Guidelines section.

No matter how you travel, it is always good to bring your nutrition guide and dining card and have your survival stash in your daypack, carry-on luggage, or in your briefcase. Pack a couple of plastic bags of trail mix, meal replacement bars, foil pouches of tuna, nuts, or crackers. If you are delayed, you will still have snacks available.

Most importantly, remember that traveling is fun! Enjoy yourself. With proper planning, you will arrive at your destination with the resources you need to have a terrific vacation!

Notes:

_____

_____

_____

_____

_____

_____

_____

_____

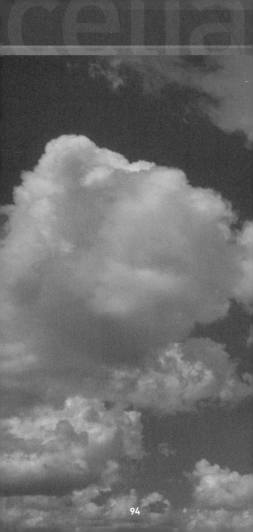

Religious Observances

A diagnosis of celiac disease is challenging enough, but the additional burden of managing a religious holiday or mass in which a wheat based product is central to the celebration adds even more stress.

For those of Jewish faith, problems arise during Passover in which the use of wheat-based matzo is central to the weeklong observances. The good news is that unleavened, gluten-free substitutes made from oats are now available. Whole Foods Market, along with many kosher markets, carries gluten-free matzo during Passover.

For those of Catholic faith, receiving the Eucharist at Mass each week may propose a challenge. Canon law states that the host used during the Eucharist must be made of wheat. Based on these grounds, the Vatican has determined that gluten-free hosts are not valid matter for the Eucharist. Since Catholic teaching holds that the whole of Christ's Body is contained in both the bread and the wine, Catholic celiacs who wish to receive the Eucharist may take Communion under the form of wine. Celiac sufferers must also keep in mind that because the priest deliberately places a piece of the host into the wine during the rite of fractions, it is not safe to drink from the priest's chalice.

The U.S. Conference of Catholic Bishops has determined that a person with Celiac disease is entitled to receive Communion from a separate cup because of issues with cross contamination from the wheat host during consecration and distribution of the Eucharist. Check with your pastor about making arrangements to safely receive Communion. Another alternative is a low gluten host developed by the Benedictine Sisters that contains less than 0.01% of gluten which is actually below what is considered gluten-free. The hosts can be obtained from the Benedictine Sisters of Perpetual Adoration.

Whether or not you feel comfortable consuming a product that is not completely gluten-free is a personal decision. According to the information we have today, the low gluten host is safe for the individual who maintains a strict gluten-free diet. For further information on this, please contact the Catholic Celiac Society.

Religious Observances

Contact Information:

Lakewood Matzoh
501 Prospect Street
Lakewood, NJ 08701
(732) 364-8757
www.lakewoodmatzoh.com

Benedictine Sisters of Perpetual Adoration
Altar Bread Department
31970 State Highway P
Clyde, MO 64432
(800) 223-2772
altarbreads@benedictinesisters.org

Catholic Celiac Society
2 Milano Court
Croton On Hudson, NY 10520
(914) 737-5291
www.catholicceliacs.org

Ener-G Communion Wafers
5960 First Avenue South
Seattle, Washington 98108
(800) 331-5222
www.ener-g.com/communion-wafers.html

Gluten-Free Challah

Everybody Eats (not Kosher)
www.everybodyeats-inc.com

Katz Gluten Free
www.katzglutenfree.com

Kosher Naturals Gluten-Free
www.glutenfreemall.com

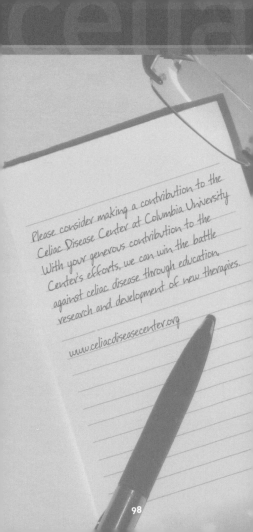

Please consider making a contribution to the
Celiac Disease Center at Columbia University
With your generous contribution to the
Center's efforts, we can win the battle
against celiac disease through education,
research and development of new therapies.

www.celiacdiseasecenter.org

The Celiac Disease Center at Columbia University Medical Center has established itself as a leader in the field, both nationally and internationally, by providing the highest quality, compassionate patient care for children and adults with celiac disease.

Our strengths in research and treatment are enhanced by our location within Columbia University Medical Center, which as a leading medical institution in New York City provides fertile ground for innovative research and translational studies across a variety of divisions, departments, centers, and institutes. As a center in the Department of Medicine at Columbia University, we are able to take advantage of many opportunities for interdisciplinary patient care and research. All of the Center's research is directed toward celiac disease and reflects the nature of celiac disease as a multisystem disorder.

Clinical research at the Center has led to studies on adults and children that describe the clinical face of celiac disease in the United States. The many research and review publications emanating from the Center are available at www.celiacdiseasecenter.org.

These activities, combined with successful treatment outcomes for our patients, have enabled the Celiac Disease Center to greatly impact the rate of diagnosis and awareness among physicians in the United States. We think advocacy in the medical community is one of the most effective ways to increase the profile and knowledge base of celiac disease to healthcare professionals. As the rate of diagnosis increases, the visibility of celiac disease will continue to grow, with physicians considering the diagnoses in greater numbers, resulting in better services for those with the disease and a markedly improved quality of life for these patients.

A Patient-Centered Approach

Using a multidisciplinary approach, the Center delivers individualized care to meet the needs of each patient. Our team consists of adult and pediatric gastroenterologists.

Services provided include:

- Medical consultation
- Nutritional assessment and counseling
- Breath testing for bacterial overgrowth and lactose, fructose and sucrose intolerance
- Endoscopy (including double balloon enteroscopy)
- Video capsule endoscopy
- Pathology
- Genetic testing

In addition, extensive collaborative relationships have been established with other medical and subspecialist departments including endocrinology, bone metabolism, rheumatology, surgery, hematology, oncology, neurology and dental medicine.

This team approach ensures that there is continuity in care, which is especially important for the youngest patients diagnosed with celiac disease. It is well known that children experience difficulty adhering to a gluten-free diet as they transition through the different developmental stages from childhood to young adulthood. Our approach ensures that each child we treat has an established relationship with a registered dietitian to supplement parental guidance at these vulnerable periods and throughout their adult lives.

Outreach and Education

One of the major roles of the Celiac Disease Center at Columbia University Medical Center is to raise awareness about celiac disease and to educate others in the medical community so that each year fewer cases go undiagnosed. In an effort to educate the public, our physicians have been featured on regional and national radio programs, television shows, and in prominent newspapers and magazines. We have also developed educational materials about celiac disease for children and adults and conduct annual educational events and family screening programs. Within the medical community, our physicians have lectured on celiac disease at many medical institutions throughout the United States as well as national and international meetings. The Center has assumed a leadership role by organizing conferences for physicians, nutritionists, and other healthcare practitioners.

Patient Advocacy

One of the important roles of the Celiac Disease Center at Columbia University Medical Center, as a leading university based Center, is patient advocacy with respect to legislative, health and life insurance and funding for all aspects of celiac disease research, education and patient management.

Cutting-Edge Research

While much is known about the origin and development of celiac disease, there is still much to be discovered. Important issues to be studied include the long-term quality of life of individuals with celiac disease, their psychological welfare, and their ability to adapt to a gluten-free diet. In addition, our laboratory is attempting to explore the mechanisms of the immunological damage in celiac disease. Looking ahead, the Center will continue to pursue pioneering research that explores the relationship of celiac disease to other autoimmune diseases with emphasis on neurological, thyroid, and cardiovascular disorders. We believe in a collaborative approach to research. Most of our studies are conducted in conjunction with experts in other medical disciplines at Columbia University Medical Center, as well as with other national and international investigators.

The Columbia University Medical Center's Biomedical research is at a critical juncture, with scientists primed to make improvements in health care that will open endless opportunities for how we treat patients and prevent disease. However, only a handful of academic medical centers possess the range of expertise, the tradition of excellence, the foresight, and the scientific innovation to translate this promise into practice. Columbia University Medical Center (CUMC) is a leader among these select institutions.

Furthermore, patients who visit CUMC benefit from access to new and innovative treatments that simply are not available outside a major research institution. Nowhere is this scientific leadership more prominent than in our efforts to study and treat celiac disease, which affects a growing number of individuals each year.

About the Center

Peter H.R. Green, M.D., has served as Director of the Celiac Disease Center at Columbia University Medical Center in the Department of Medicine since 2001 and is one of a few recognized experts on celiac disease in the United States. Dr. Green's excellence in the field is widely recognized, and his work has positioned Columbia at the forefront of national and international scholarship on the diagnosis, treatment and research of celiac disease.

The Celiac Disease Center at Columbia University Medical Center has long been active in physician education on celiac disease in order to increase the rate of diagnosis.

About the Center

Defining the Future of Celiac Disease

Columbia University Medical Center and its Department of Medicine are strongly committed to the mission of the Celiac Disease Center and its program to deliver the highest-quality care, access to the latest therapies, and innovative research from an experienced, compassionate, and multi-disciplinary team.

Already a leading Center for celiac disease research, treatment, and education in the nation, we are poised to build an even stronger and expanded program that will serve as a model for other institutions. We hope that you will partner with us to continue the excellent care, innovative research, and education that will improve the lives of so many people suffering from celiac disease.

An Invitation

The Celiac Disease Center at Columbia University Medical Center could not have been established nor would it exist today without the generosity of many individuals. The Center continues to depend upon major gifts to continue its vital work on the leading edge of research, treatment, education and advocacy.

If you would like to share in the effort to insure a better life for celiac patients, we invite you to join our generous friends in donating to the Center. For more information, please visit us online at www.celiacdiseasecenter.org. With your contribution to the Center's efforts, we can win the battle against celiac disease through education, research and development of new therapies.

Donate Online

Please visit us online at www.celiacdisease-center.org to use our convenient form to donate online using a credit card. Please make your check payable to Trustees of Columbia University and mail to:

Celiac Disease Center at Columbia
University Medical Center
Harkness Pavilion
180 Fort Washington Avenue
Suite 934
New York, NY 10032

The Celiac Disease Center at Columbia University Medical Center is a 501(c)(3) non-profit organization. The (Columbia University) EIN number is 13-5598093.

Celiac Disease Center at Columbia
University Medical Center
Harkness Pavilion
180 Fort Washington Avenue
Suite 934
New York, NY 10032
(212) 342-4529
cb2280@ columbia.edu

www.celiacdiseasecenter.org

Center Team

Adult Gastroenterology

Peter H. R. Green, MD
Professor of Clinical Medicine
Director, Celiac Disease Center at Columbia
University Medical Center
(212) 305-5590

Benjamin Lebwohl, MD
Assistant Professor of Clinical Medicine and
Clinical Epidemiology
(212) 305-5590

Suzanne K. Lewis, MD
Associate Professor of Clinical Medicine
(212) 305-5590

Christina Tennyson, MD
Assistant Professor of Clinical Medicine
(212) 305-5590

Pediatric Gastroenterology

Amy R. DeFelice, MD
Professor of Pediatrics
(212) 305-5903

Philip G. Kazlow, MD
Professor of Pediatrics
(212) 305-5903

Norelle Rizkalla Reilly
Assistant Professor of Clinical Pediatrics
(212) 305-5903

Nutrition

Suzanne Simpson, RD
Clinical Nutritionist
(212) 305-5590

Development, Education & Patient Advocacy

Cynthia Beckman
Director of Development
(212) 342-4529
email: cb2280@columbia.edu